FROM SEED TO PLATE

COOKBOOK

20 Fresh, Delicious And Nutritious Diet Recipes for Breast Cancer Resilience Patients For A Healthy Lifestyle.

MARIYAM MOHL

Acknowledgment

I'd want to express my gratitude to everyone who contributed to the creation of this book.

First and foremost, I'd want to thank the cancer patients and survivors who have shared their stories and ideas with me, inspiring me to write this book. Your courage, tenacity, and dedication are an inspiration to us all.

Foreword

As a healthcare professional and cancer survivor, I've seen personally how a cancer diagnosis may affect a person's physical, emotional, and mental well-being. Cancer treatment may be a difficult and exhausting process; therefore it is critical to develop ways to support recovery and well-being.

Dedication

This book is dedicated to all cancer patients and survivors who have faced the challenges of cancer treatment and recovery with bravery, resilience, and determination.

Your tenacity and endurance have inspired me and countless others. It is my hope that this book will provide you with practical knowledge and guidance on how to include gardening into your cancer treatment and recovery process, as well as help you discover healing, wellness, and joy in nature.

TABLE OF CONTENT

INTRODUCTION

Nutrition is an important ally on the path to breast cancer resistance. The marriage of colorful, nutrient-dense foods with the artistry of culinary creation creates a potent road to healing and well-being.

"From Seed to Plate Cookbook: Recipes for Breast Cancer Resilience" is more than just a cookbook; it's a personal investigation of the inextricable link between food, wellness, and empowerment.

Within these pages, you'll find a symphony of tastes that have been painstakingly handpicked to not only delight your taste senses but also to fortify your body.

Every ingredient is picked with care, and each recipe is designed to maximize the natural power of nature's wealth. From the lush soil of the garden to the warmth of your plate, this collection invites you to embark on a nourishing journey that goes beyond the kitchen—a journey toward resilience and vitality.

These dishes are more than culinary masterpieces; they are acts of love and unity as they go on a quest to help individuals managing the hardships of breast cancer. Each dish is proof that every mouthful may be a step towards regeneration and rejuvenation. These dishes become partners in your pursuit of well-being through deliberate blends of cancer-fighting superfoods, antioxidants, and immune-boosting components.

"From Seed to Plate Cookbook" is a companion on your route to health and vitality, whether you are seeking comfort in the kitchen, discovering new flavors, or looking for methods to better your nutritional journey. Each recipe is a celebration of life, tenacity, and the everlasting inner strength.

Here's to sustenance, healing, and the enlightening journey from garden to plate.

Chia Seed Pudding with Berries

Ingredients:
- 1/4 cup chia seeds
- 1 cup almond milk
- Mixed berries (strawberries, blueberries, raspberries)
- Honey for sweetness (optional)

Instructions:
1. In a bowl, combine chia seeds and almond milk.
2. Stir well to ensure the chia seeds are evenly distributed in the almond milk.
3. Let the mixture sit for about 15 minutes, stirring occasionally to prevent clumping.
4. Cover the bowl and refrigerate for at least 2 hours or overnight to allow the chia seeds to absorb the liquid and create a pudding-like consistency.
5. Before serving, stir the pudding to break up any clumps and achieve a smooth texture.
6. Top the chia seed pudding with an assortment of mixed berries.
7. Drizzle honey over the pudding if additional sweetness is desired.

Benefits:

- **Omega-3 Fatty Acids:** Chia seeds are rich in omega-3 fatty acids, which contribute to heart health and reduce inflammation.
- **Fiber:** Chia seeds are an excellent source of fiber, promoting digestive health and aiding in weight management.
- **Antioxidants:** Berries are packed with antioxidants, which help protect cells from damage caused by free radicals.
- **Protein:** Chia seeds contain a decent amount of protein, making this pudding a satisfying and nutritious snack.
- **Vitamins and Minerals:** Almond milk adds essential nutrients like vitamin E and calcium to the pudding.

Application:

- **Breakfast:** Enjoy this chia seed pudding with berries as a healthy and energizing breakfast option.
- **Snack:** Serve the pudding as a midday snack to curb cravings and boost nutrient intake.
- **Dessert:** As a wholesome dessert, the natural sweetness from berries and optional honey makes it a guilt-free treat.
- **Post-Workout:** The combination of protein, fiber, and antioxidants makes it a

suitable post-workout snack for muscle recovery and overall well-being.

Kale and Pomegranate Smoothie

Ingredients:
- 1 cup kale leaves, stems removed
- 1/2 cup pomegranate seeds
- 1 ripe banana
- 1 cup almond milk
- Ice cubes (optional)

Instructions:
1. Wash the kale leaves thoroughly, removing the stems.
2. In a blender, combine kale leaves, pomegranate seeds, banana, and almond milk.
3. Blend until smooth and creamy. Add ice cubes if a colder consistency is desired.
4. Pour the smoothie into a glass and garnish with a few extra pomegranate seeds for texture.

Benefits:
- **Vitamins and Minerals:** Kale is a nutrient powerhouse, providing vitamins A, C, and K, as well as minerals like calcium and potassium.

- **Antioxidants:** Pomegranate seeds are rich in antioxidants, which help combat oxidative stress and inflammation in the body.
- **Fiber:** Both kale and pomegranate contribute to the smoothie's fiber content, promoting digestive health.
- **Energy Boost:** The natural sugars from the banana and pomegranate provide a quick and healthy energy boost.
- **Hydration:** Almond milk adds a hydrating element to the smoothie, contributing to overall fluid intake.

Application:

- **Breakfast:** Start your day with this nutrient-packed smoothie for a refreshing and energizing breakfast.
- **Post-Workout:** The combination of carbohydrates, vitamins, and minerals makes it an excellent choice for post-exercise recovery.
- **Snack:** Enjoy the smoothie as a wholesome and satisfying snack between meals.
- **Detox:** Incorporate this smoothie into a detox routine, thanks to the cleansing properties of kale and the antioxidants in pomegranate.
- **Customization:** Experiment with additional ingredients such as chia seeds,

Greek yogurt, or a touch of honey to tailor the smoothie to your taste preferences.

Rosemary Roasted Chicken Thighs

Ingredients:
- 4 bone-in, skin-on chicken thighs
- 2 tablespoons olive oil
- 3 cloves garlic, minced
- 1 tablespoon fresh rosemary, finely chopped
- 1 teaspoon salt
- 1/2 teaspoon black pepper
- Juice of 1 lemon

Instructions:
1. Preheat the oven to 400°F (200°C).
2. In a small bowl, mix together olive oil, minced garlic, chopped rosemary, salt, and black pepper.
3. Pat the chicken thighs dry with paper towels and place them in a roasting pan.
4. Rub the olive oil mixture over each chicken thigh, ensuring they are well coated.
5. Squeeze the lemon juice over the chicken thighs for a burst of citrus flavor.
6. Roast in the preheated oven for 35-40 minutes or until the chicken reaches an

internal temperature of 165°F (74°C) and the skin is golden and crispy.

7. Allow the chicken to rest for a few minutes before serving.

Benefits:

- **Protein:** Chicken thighs are a good source of lean protein, essential for muscle growth and repair.
- **Healthy Fats:** Olive oil provides healthy monounsaturated fats, promoting heart health.
- **Rosemary:** Contains antioxidants and anti-inflammatory compounds, potentially offering health benefits.
- **Garlic:** Known for its immune-boosting properties and potential cardiovascular benefits.
- **Vitamin C:** Lemon juice contributes vitamin C, supporting immune function.

Application:

- **Main Course:** Serve the Rosemary Roasted Chicken Thighs as the centerpiece of a wholesome dinner.
- **Meal Prep:** Prepare a batch and use the roasted chicken thighs in meal prep for the week.
- **Family Gatherings:** Ideal for family dinners or gatherings, as the aroma of rosemary adds a comforting touch.

- **Salads:** Shred the roasted chicken and add it to salads for a protein-packed, flavorful twist.
- **Versatility:** Pair with your favorite side dishes such as roasted vegetables, quinoa, or a fresh green salad.

Mango and Black Bean Quinoa Salad

Ingredients:
- 1 cup quinoa, rinsed
- 2 cups water
- 1 ripe mango, diced
- 1 can (15 oz) black beans, drained and rinsed
- 1 red bell pepper, diced
- 1/4 cup red onion, finely chopped
- 1/4 cup fresh cilantro, chopped
- Juice of 2 limes
- 2 tablespoons olive oil
- Salt and pepper to taste

Instructions:
1. In a medium saucepan, bring 2 cups of water to a boil. Add quinoa, reduce heat to low, cover, and simmer for 15-20 minutes or until water is absorbed and quinoa is cooked. Fluff with a fork and let it cool.

2. In a large bowl, combine cooked quinoa, diced mango, black beans, red bell pepper, red onion, and cilantro.
3. In a small bowl, whisk together lime juice, olive oil, salt, and pepper.
4. Pour the dressing over the quinoa mixture and toss gently to coat evenly.
5. Refrigerate for at least 30 minutes to allow the flavors to meld.
6. Serve chilled, garnished with additional cilantro if desired.

Benefits:

- **Quinoa:** A complete protein source, rich in fiber, and various vitamins and minerals.
- **Mango:** Packed with vitamins A and C, antioxidants, and adds natural sweetness.
- **Black Beans:** Excellent source of plant-based protein, fiber, and essential nutrients.
- **Bell Pepper:** High in vitamin C and adds a crunch to the salad.
- **Cilantro:** Provides fresh flavor and contains antioxidants.

Application:

- **Lunch or Dinner:** Enjoy the Mango and Black Bean Quinoa Salad as a light and satisfying lunch or dinner.

- **Side Dish:** Serve as a refreshing side dish at barbecues or potlucks.
- **Meal Prep:** Perfect for meal prep, as it can be stored in the fridge for several days.
- **Taco Filling:** Use the salad as a delicious and nutritious filling for tacos or wraps.
- **Picnics and Outdoor Events:** Portable and vibrant, making it an excellent choice for picnics and outdoor gatherings.

Eggplant and Tomato Bake

Ingredients:
- 2 medium-sized eggplants, sliced
- 3 large tomatoes, sliced
- 1 cup mozzarella cheese, shredded
- 1/4 cup fresh basil, chopped
- 2 cloves garlic, minced
- 2 tablespoons olive oil
- Salt and pepper to taste
- Parmesan cheese for topping (optional)

Instructions:
1. Preheat the oven to 375°F (190°C).
2. Place eggplant slices on a baking sheet and brush both sides with olive oil. Sprinkle with salt and pepper.
3. Bake the eggplant slices for 15-20 minutes or until they become tender.

Remove from the oven and let them cool slightly.

4. In a separate bowl, mix together minced garlic and chopped basil.
5. In a baking dish, layer the eggplant slices, tomato slices, and sprinkle with the garlic and basil mixture.
6. Repeat the layering until all ingredients are used, finishing with a layer of tomatoes on top.
7. Sprinkle mozzarella cheese evenly over the top.
8. Bake in the preheated oven for 25-30 minutes or until the cheese is melted and bubbly.
9. If desired, sprinkle Parmesan cheese on top during the last 5 minutes of baking.
10. Remove from the oven, let it cool slightly, and serve.

Benefits:
- **Eggplant:** Rich in fiber, vitamins, and minerals, and contains antioxidants that support heart health.
- **Tomatoes:** High in vitamins C and K, as well as antioxidants like lycopene, known for its potential health benefits.
- **Mozzarella Cheese:** Provides calcium and protein, essential for bone health and muscle function.

- **Basil and Garlic:** Both add flavor and contain antioxidants with potential health-promoting properties.
- **Olive Oil:** Healthy monounsaturated fats support heart health.

Application:

- **Main Dish:** Serve as a flavorful vegetarian main dish.
- **Side Dish:** Complement your protein of choice with a serving of Eggplant and Tomato Bake.
- **Appetizer:** Cut into smaller portions for a delicious appetizer at gatherings.
- **Meal Prep:** Prepare ahead and reheat for a quick and nutritious meal during busy days.
- **Mediterranean Cuisine:** Pair with a side of couscous or quinoa for a Mediterranean-inspired meal.

Cucumber and Dill Yogurt Dip

Ingredients:

- 1 cup Greek yogurt
- 1 cucumber, finely diced
- 2 tablespoons fresh dill, finely chopped
- 1 clove garlic, minced
- 1 tablespoon lemon juice
- Salt and pepper to taste

Instructions:

1. In a bowl, combine Greek yogurt, diced cucumber, chopped dill, minced garlic, and lemon juice.
2. Mix the ingredients thoroughly to ensure an even distribution of flavors.
3. Season the dip with salt and pepper to taste.
4. Refrigerate for at least 30 minutes to allow the flavors to meld.
5. Before serving, garnish with additional fresh dill for a burst of color and flavor.
6. Serve chilled with your favorite dippable.

Benefits:

- **Greek Yogurt:** A good source of protein, probiotics, and calcium, supporting gut health and bone strength.
- **Cucumber:** Hydrating and low in calories, adds a refreshing crunch to the dip.
- **Dill:** Rich in antioxidants and adds a fresh, aromatic flavor.
- **Garlic:** Known for its potential immune-boosting and anti-inflammatory properties.
- **Lemon Juice:** Adds a zesty brightness while providing vitamin C.

Application:

- **Vegetable Dip:** Serve with a variety of fresh vegetables such as carrots, bell peppers, and cherry tomatoes.
- **Pita Bread or Chips:** Enjoy as a dip with toasted pita bread or pita chips.
- **Grilled Meats:** Pair with grilled chicken, lamb, or kebabs for a flavorful accompaniment.
- **Sandwich Spread:** Use as a spread for sandwiches or wraps.
- **Salad Dressing Base:** Thin with a bit of water to create a refreshing dressing for salads.

Brussels Sprouts and Walnut Salad

Ingredients:

- 1 lb Brussels sprouts, trimmed and thinly sliced
- 1 cup walnuts, toasted and roughly chopped
- 1/2 cup dried cranberries
- 1/4 cup Parmesan cheese, shaved
- 2 tablespoons olive oil
- 2 tablespoons balsamic vinegar
- 1 tablespoon Dijon mustard
- Salt and pepper to taste

Instructions:

1. In a large bowl, combine the thinly sliced Brussels sprouts, toasted walnuts, dried cranberries, and Parmesan cheese.
2. In a separate small bowl, whisk together olive oil, balsamic vinegar, Dijon mustard, salt, and pepper to create the dressing.
3. Pour the dressing over the Brussels sprouts mixture and toss well to ensure even coating.
4. Allow the salad to sit for 10-15 minutes before serving to let the flavors meld.
5. Just before serving, toss the salad again and adjust the seasoning if necessary.
6. Garnish with additional shaved Parmesan if desired.

Benefits:

- **Brussels Sprouts:** Rich in fiber, vitamins C and K, and antioxidants that may promote heart health.
- **Walnuts:** High in omega-3 fatty acids, antioxidants, and provide a satisfying crunch.
- **Dried Cranberries:** Add sweetness and are a good source of vitamins and antioxidants.
- **Parmesan Cheese:** Adds a savory depth of flavor and contributes calcium and protein.

- **Olive Oil:** Contains healthy monounsaturated fats, supporting heart health.
- **Balsamic Vinegar:** Provides a tangy acidity and potential health benefits.

Application:

- **Side Dish:** Serve as a vibrant and nutritious side dish alongside grilled meats or roasted vegetables.
- **Lunch Salad:** Enjoy a hearty portion as a standalone lunch salad.
- **Potluck or Gathering:** Bring to potlucks or gatherings for a colorful and flavorful contribution.
- **Holiday Meal:** A festive addition to holiday feasts, offering a balance of flavors and textures.
- **Meal Prep:** Prepare ahead for a quick and satisfying lunch option throughout the week.

Garlic and Herb Baked Cod

Ingredients:

- 4 cod fillets
- 3 tablespoons olive oil
- 4 cloves garlic, minced
- 1 tablespoon fresh parsley, chopped
- 1 tablespoon fresh dill, chopped

- 1 lemon, sliced
- Salt and pepper to taste

Instructions:

1. Preheat the oven to 400°F (200°C).
2. Place the cod fillets in a baking dish lined with parchment paper.
3. In a small bowl, mix together olive oil, minced garlic, chopped parsley, chopped dill, salt, and pepper.
4. Brush the cod fillets with the herb and garlic mixture, ensuring they are well coated.
5. Place lemon slices on top of each fillet for added flavor.
6. Bake in the preheated oven for 15-20 minutes or until the cod is opaque and flakes easily with a fork.
7. If desired, broil for an additional 2-3 minutes to achieve a golden crust.
8. Garnish with extra herbs and serve with lemon wedges.

Benefits:

- **Cod:** A lean source of protein, rich in omega-3 fatty acids, and provides essential vitamins and minerals.
- **Olive Oil:** Healthy monounsaturated fats, contributing to heart health.

- **Garlic:** Known for its potential immune-boosting properties and adds savory depth to the dish.
- **Fresh Herbs:** Parsley and dill provide flavor and contain antioxidants with potential health benefits.
- **Lemon:** Adds a burst of citrus flavor and provides vitamin C.

Application:

- **Main Course:** Serve the Garlic and Herb Baked Cod as the centerpiece of a light and healthy main course.
- **Low-Carb Meal:** Ideal for those following a low-carb or keto diet.
- **Meal Prep:** Prepare a batch for meal prep and enjoy throughout the week.
- **Seafood Night:** Perfect for a themed seafood dinner paired with your favorite side dishes.
- **Special Occasions:** Impress guests with this flavorful and visually appealing dish for special occasions.

Brown Rice and Black Bean Bowl

Ingredients:

- 1 cup brown rice
- 2 cups water or vegetable broth

- 1 can (15 oz) black beans, drained and rinsed
- 1 cup corn kernels (fresh, frozen, or canned)
- 1 red bell pepper, diced
- 1 avocado, sliced
- Fresh cilantro, chopped (for garnish)
- Lime wedges (for serving)

Instructions:

1. Rinse the brown rice under cold water. In a saucepan, combine the brown rice and water or vegetable broth. Bring to a boil, then reduce the heat to low, cover, and simmer for 40-45 minutes or until the rice is tender and water is absorbed.
2. In a separate pot, heat the black beans and corn until warmed through.
3. Dice the red bell pepper and slice the avocado.
4. Assemble the bowl by dividing the cooked brown rice among serving bowls. Top with black beans, corn, diced red bell pepper, and avocado slices.
5. Garnish with fresh cilantro and serve with lime wedges on the side for squeezing over the bowl.

Benefits:

- **Brown Rice:** Rich in fiber, vitamins, and minerals, providing sustained energy and supporting digestive health.
- **Black Beans:** Excellent source of plant-based protein, fiber, and essential nutrients.
- **Corn:** Adds natural sweetness and provides vitamins, minerals, and antioxidants.
- **Red Bell Pepper:** High in vitamin C and adds crunch and vibrant color to the bowl.
- **Avocado:** Loaded with healthy monounsaturated fats, vitamins, and minerals.
- **Cilantro:** Adds a burst of fresh flavor and contains antioxidants.

Application:

- **Main Dish:** Enjoy the Brown Rice and Black Bean Bowl as a wholesome and satisfying main course.
- **Meal Prep:** Perfect for weekly meal prep, as it can be portioned into containers for easy grab-and-go lunches.
- **Burrito Bowl:** Use the components as a filling for a burrito or taco bowl.
- **Vegan Option:** Skip the animal products for a hearty and nutritious vegan meal.
- **Customization:** Add salsa, Greek yogurt, or your favorite hot sauce for extra flavor.

Avocado and Grapefruit Salad

Ingredients:

- 2 ripe avocados, sliced
- 2 pink grapefruits, segmented
- Mixed salad greens (e.g., arugula, spinach, or watercress)
- 1/4 cup red onion, thinly sliced
- 1/4 cup fresh mint leaves, chopped
- 2 tablespoons extra-virgin olive oil
- 1 tablespoon balsamic vinegar
- Salt and pepper to taste

Instructions:

1. In a large bowl, combine the sliced avocados, segmented grapefruits, mixed salad greens, sliced red onion, and chopped mint leaves.
2. In a small bowl, whisk together the olive oil and balsamic vinegar to create the dressing.
3. Drizzle the dressing over the salad and gently toss to combine.
4. Season with salt and pepper to taste.
5. Allow the salad to sit for a few minutes to let the flavors meld.
6. Serve chilled, garnished with additional mint leaves if desired.

Benefits:

- **Avocado:** Packed with healthy monounsaturated fats, vitamins, and minerals.
- **Grapefruit:** Rich in vitamin C, antioxidants, and may aid in weight management.
- **Salad Greens:** Provide fiber, vitamins, and minerals while adding freshness and crunch.
- **Red Onion:** Adds a mild, sweet flavor and contains antioxidants.
- **Mint:** Adds a refreshing element and may aid in digestion.
- **Olive Oil:** Healthy monounsaturated fats with potential heart health benefits.

Application:

- **Side Dish:** Serve as a vibrant and refreshing side dish alongside grilled proteins or other main courses.
- **Lunch Salad:** Enjoy a generous portion as a standalone lunch salad.
- **Brunch:** A delightful addition to brunch, pairing well with a variety of dishes.
- **Picnic or Potluck:** Portable and visually appealing, making it suitable for outdoor gatherings.
- **Summer Entertaining:** Perfect for summer entertaining, offering a light and flavorful option.

Zucchini and Carrot Ribbon Salad

Ingredients

- 2 medium-sized zucchinis
- 2 large carrots
- 1/4 cup olive oil
- 2 tablespoons balsamic vinegar
- 1 clove garlic, minced
- 1 tablespoon Dijon mustard
- Salt and pepper to taste
- Fresh basil or parsley for garnish (optional)

Instructions:

1. Using a vegetable peeler or a mandoline, create thin ribbons of zucchini and carrots. Place them in a large salad bowl.
2. In a small bowl, whisk together olive oil, balsamic vinegar, minced garlic, Dijon mustard, salt, and pepper to create the dressing.
3. Pour the dressing over the zucchini and carrot ribbons.
4. Gently toss the salad to ensure even coating of the vegetables with the dressing.
5. Allow the salad to marinate for at least 15 minutes to let the flavors meld.
6. Garnish with fresh basil or parsley just before serving.

7. Serve chilled.

Benefits:
- **Zucchini:** Low in calories, a good source of fiber, vitamins A and C, and antioxidants.
- **Carrots:** Packed with beta-carotene, vitamins, and minerals, promoting eye health and immune function.
- **Olive Oil:** Healthy monounsaturated fats supporting heart health.
- **Balsamic Vinegar:** Adds a sweet and tangy flavor, and may have potential health benefits.
- **Garlic:** Known for its immune-boosting properties and adds savory depth.
- **Dijon Mustard:** Adds a zesty kick and is low in calories.

Application:
- **Side Dish:** Serve as a light and refreshing side dish with grilled chicken, fish, or as part of a picnic spread.
- **Summer BBQ:** Complement grilled meats with the vibrant colors and flavors of this salad.
- **Lunch or Dinner Salad:** Enjoy a larger portion as a standalone salad for a light lunch or dinner.

- **Potluck or Gathering:** A visually appealing dish that's easy to transport and share.
- **Meal Prep:** Prepare ahead and refrigerate for quick and healthy lunches throughout the week.

Whole Grain Pasta with Tomato and Basil Sauce

Ingredients:

- 8 oz whole grain pasta (such as whole wheat or quinoa pasta)
- 2 tablespoons olive oil
- 3 cloves garlic, minced
- 1 can (28 oz) crushed tomatoes
- 1 teaspoon dried oregano
- 1 teaspoon dried basil
- Salt and pepper to taste
- Fresh basil leaves, chopped, for garnish
- Grated Parmesan cheese (optional)

Instructions:

1. Cook the whole grain pasta according to package instructions in a pot of salted boiling water. Drain and set aside.
2. In a large saucepan, heat olive oil over medium heat. Add minced garlic and sauté until fragrant, about 1-2 minutes.

3. Pour in the crushed tomatoes and add dried oregano, dried basil, salt, and pepper. Stir to combine.
4. Simmer the sauce over low heat for 15-20 minutes to allow the flavors to meld.
5. Adjust salt and pepper to taste. If the sauce is too thick, you can add a splash of water to achieve your desired consistency.
6. Toss the cooked pasta into the tomato and basil sauce, ensuring the pasta is well coated.
7. Serve the pasta in bowls, garnished with fresh chopped basil and grated Parmesan cheese if desired.

Benefits:

- **Whole Grain Pasta:** Higher in fiber and nutrients compared to refined pasta, contributing to digestive health and satiety.
- **Olive Oil:** Provides healthy monounsaturated fats, supporting heart health.
- **Garlic:** Adds flavor and may have potential health benefits, including immune support.
- **Tomatoes:** Rich in vitamins, antioxidants, and lycopene, supporting overall health.

- **Basil:** Contains antioxidants and adds a fresh, aromatic flavor.

Application:

- **Quick Dinner:** Perfect for a quick and satisfying weeknight dinner.
- **Lunch Prep:** Prepare a batch for meal prep to enjoy throughout the week.
- **Vegetarian Dish:** A delicious and nutritious option for vegetarians.
- **Family-Friendly Meal:** Loved by both adults and kids alike.
- **Pair with Salad:** Serve alongside a fresh green salad for a complete meal.

Garlic and Rosemary Roasted Sweet Potatoes

Ingredients:

- 4 medium-sized sweet potatoes, peeled and diced
- 3 tablespoons olive oil
- 4 cloves garlic, minced
- 1 tablespoon fresh rosemary, finely chopped
- Salt and black pepper to taste

Instructions:

1. Preheat the oven to 400°F (200°C).

2. In a large bowl, toss the diced sweet potatoes with olive oil, minced garlic, chopped rosemary, salt, and black pepper.
3. Spread the seasoned sweet potatoes evenly on a baking sheet lined with parchment paper.
4. Roast in the preheated oven for 25-30 minutes or until the sweet potatoes are tender and golden brown, turning them halfway through for even cooking.
5. Remove from the oven and let them rest for a few minutes before serving.

Benefits:

- **Sweet Potatoes:** Rich in vitamins A and C, fiber, and antioxidants, supporting immune health and digestion.
- **Olive Oil:** Provides healthy monounsaturated fats, promoting heart health.
- **Garlic:** Adds flavor and potential immune-boosting properties.
- **Rosemary:** Contains antioxidants and anti-inflammatory compounds.
- **Black Pepper:** May enhance nutrient absorption and digestion.

Application:

- **Side Dish:** Serve as a flavorful side dish alongside grilled chicken, fish, or your favorite protein.
- **Holiday Meal:** A delicious addition to holiday feasts, offering a healthier alternative to traditional sides.
- **Meal Prep:** Prepare a batch for meal prep and use throughout the week.
- **Vegetarian Bowl:** Incorporate into vegetarian bowls or wraps for added flavor and nutrients.
- **Snack:** Enjoy as a nutritious and satisfying snack on its own.

Lentil and Vegetable Curry

Ingredients:

- 1 cup dry green or brown lentils, rinsed
- 2 tablespoons vegetable oil
- 1 large onion, finely chopped
- 3 cloves garlic, minced
- 1 tablespoon ginger, grated
- 2 tablespoons curry powder
- 1 teaspoon ground cumin
- 1 teaspoon ground coriander
- 1 teaspoon turmeric
- 1 can (14 oz) diced tomatoes
- 1 can (14 oz) coconut milk

- 3 cups mixed vegetables (e.g., carrots, bell peppers, peas)
- Salt and pepper to taste
- Fresh cilantro, chopped (for garnish)
- Cooked rice or naan bread (for serving)

Instructions:

1. Cook the lentils according to package instructions. Drain and set aside.
2. In a large pot, heat the vegetable oil over medium heat. Add chopped onions and cook until softened.
3. Add minced garlic and grated ginger to the onions, cooking for an additional 2 minutes until fragrant.
4. Stir in curry powder, ground cumin, ground coriander, and turmeric. Cook for 1-2 minutes to toast the spices.
5. Pour in the diced tomatoes and coconut milk. Stir to combine.
6. Add the cooked lentils and mixed vegetables to the pot. Season with salt and pepper.
7. Bring the curry to a simmer and let it cook for 15-20 minutes until the vegetables are tender and the flavors meld.
8. Adjust the seasoning as needed. If the curry is too thick, you can add a bit of water.
9. Serve the Lentil and Vegetable Curry over cooked rice or with naan bread.

10. Garnish with chopped cilantro before serving.

Benefits:

- **Lentils:** High in protein, fiber, and various nutrients, promoting heart health and aiding digestion.
- **Vegetables:** Packed with vitamins, minerals, and antioxidants, supporting overall health.
- **Coconut Milk:** Adds creaminess and provides healthy fats.
- **Spices (Curry, Cumin, Coriander, Turmeric):** Contribute to flavor and may have anti-inflammatory and antioxidant properties.

Application:

- **Main Course:** Serve as a flavorful vegetarian main course, paired with rice or bread.
- **Meal Prep:** Prepare a large batch for meal prep, storing in individual containers for convenient lunches or dinners.
- **Potluck or Gathering:** A crowd-pleaser for potlucks or gatherings, especially for those with dietary preferences.
- **Freezer-Friendly:** Freeze portions for future quick and easy meals.

- **Customization:** Adjust the level of spice and experiment with additional vegetables or legumes for variety.

Cauliflower and Turmeric Soup

Ingredients:
- 1 large cauliflower, chopped into florets
- 1 onion, diced
- 3 cloves garlic, minced
- 1 tablespoon fresh ginger, grated
- 1 teaspoon ground turmeric
- 1 teaspoon ground cumin
- 4 cups vegetable broth
- 1 can (14 oz) coconut milk
- 2 tablespoons olive oil
- Salt and pepper to taste
- Fresh cilantro or parsley for garnish (optional)

Instructions:
1. In a large pot, heat olive oil over medium heat. Add diced onions and cook until softened.
2. Add minced garlic and grated ginger, cooking for an additional 2 minutes until fragrant.
3. Stir in ground turmeric and ground cumin, allowing the spices to toast for about 1-2 minutes.

4. Add cauliflower florets to the pot and coat them with the spice mixture.
5. Pour in vegetable broth and bring the mixture to a boil. Reduce the heat to simmer and cook until the cauliflower is tender.
6. Use an immersion blender to blend the soup until smooth. If you don't have an immersion blender, carefully transfer the mixture to a blender in batches.
7. Stir in coconut milk and continue to simmer for an additional 5-7 minutes.
8. Season with salt and pepper to taste.
9. Serve the Cauliflower and Turmeric Soup hot, garnished with fresh cilantro or parsley if desired.

Benefits:

- **Cauliflower:** Low in calories, high in fiber, and rich in vitamins C and K.
- **Turmeric:** Contains curcumin, known for its anti-inflammatory and antioxidant properties.
- **Cumin:** Adds a warm and earthy flavor, and may aid in digestion.
- **Coconut Milk:** Adds creaminess and provides healthy fats.
- **Ginger:** Adds a zesty flavor and may have anti-inflammatory and digestive benefits.

Application:

- **Light Lunch or Dinner:** Enjoy a bowl of this soup as a light and nutritious meal.
- **Appetizer:** Serve smaller portions as an appetizer before a main course.
- **Meal Prep:** Make a large batch for meal prep, storing individual servings in the fridge or freezer.
- **Soothing Dish:** Ideal for days when you crave a comforting, warming dish.
- **Vegan and Gluten-Free Option:** Suitable for those with dietary preferences or restrictions.

Spinach and Feta Stuffed Mushrooms:

Ingredients:

- 20 large mushrooms, cleaned and stems removed
- 2 cups fresh spinach, chopped
- 1/2 cup feta cheese, crumbled
- 1/4 cup breadcrumbs
- 2 cloves garlic, minced
- 2 tablespoons olive oil
- Salt and pepper to taste
- Fresh parsley, chopped (for garnish)

Instructions:

1. Preheat the oven to 375°F (190°C).

2. In a skillet, heat olive oil over medium heat. Add minced garlic and sauté for 1-2 minutes until fragrant.
3. Add chopped spinach to the skillet and cook until wilted, about 2-3 minutes.
4. In a bowl, combine the sautéed spinach, feta cheese, breadcrumbs, salt, and pepper. Mix well to create the stuffing.
5. Stuff each mushroom cap with the spinach and feta mixture, pressing it down slightly.
6. Place the stuffed mushrooms on a baking sheet lined with parchment paper.
7. Bake in the preheated oven for 15-20 minutes or until the mushrooms are tender and the filling is golden brown.
8. Garnish with chopped fresh parsley before serving.

Benefits:
- **Mushrooms:** Low in calories, a good source of protein, and rich in vitamins and minerals.
- **Spinach:** Packed with iron, vitamins A and K, and antioxidants.
- **Feta Cheese:** Adds a creamy texture and provides calcium and protein.
- **Olive Oil:** Healthy monounsaturated fats, contributing to heart health.
- **Garlic:** Adds flavor and may have immune-boosting properties.

Application:

- **Appetizer:** Serve as a delightful appetizer for parties or gatherings.
- **Side Dish:** Complement a main course with these flavorful stuffed mushrooms.
- **Vegetarian Option:** A tasty vegetarian option for those looking for meat-free alternatives.
- **Snack:** Enjoy as a satisfying and nutritious snack.
- **Brunch or Breakfast:** Serve alongside other brunch items for a flavorful breakfast.

Salmon with Berry Salsa

Ingredients:

- 4 salmon fillets
- 1 cup mixed berries (such as strawberries, blueberries, and raspberries), diced
- 1/2 red onion, finely chopped
- 1 jalapeño, seeded and minced
- 1/4 cup fresh cilantro, chopped
- Juice of 1 lime
- 1 tablespoon honey or maple syrup
- Salt and pepper to taste
- 2 tablespoons olive oil

Instructions:

1. Preheat the oven to 375°F (190°C).
2. Season the salmon fillets with salt and pepper.
3. In a bowl, combine the diced berries, chopped red onion, minced jalapeño, cilantro, lime juice, honey or maple syrup, salt, and pepper. Mix well to create the berry salsa.
4. Heat olive oil in an oven-safe skillet over medium-high heat.
5. Place the seasoned salmon fillets in the skillet, skin side down, and sear for 2-3 minutes until the skin is crispy.
6. Spoon a generous amount of the berry salsa over the salmon fillets.
7. Transfer the skillet to the preheated oven and bake for 10-12 minutes or until the salmon is cooked to your liking.
8. Remove from the oven, spoon more salsa over the top, and serve.

Benefits:

- **Salmon:** Rich in omega-3 fatty acids, high-quality protein, and essential nutrients that support heart and brain health.
- **Berries:** Packed with antioxidants, vitamins, and fiber, promoting overall health.

- **Red Onion:** Adds flavor and contains antioxidants.
- **Jalapeño:** Adds a spicy kick and may have metabolism-boosting properties.
- **Cilantro:** Provides a burst of fresh flavor and contains antioxidants.
- **Olive Oil:** Healthy monounsaturated fats supporting heart health.
- **Lime:** Adds acidity and provides vitamin C.

Application:

- **Main Course:** Serve Salmon with Berry Salsa as a vibrant and flavorful main course.
- **Summer Entertaining:** Impress guests with this visually appealing dish at summer gatherings.
- **Date Night Dinner:** Perfect for a special and romantic dinner at home.
- **Grilled Variation:** Grill the salmon for a smoky flavor before topping with the berry salsa.
- **Meal Prep:** Prepare extra berry salsa to enjoy with other proteins or as a topping for salads.

Broccoli and Almond Stir-Fry

Ingredients:

- 1 lb broccoli florets
- 1 cup sliced almonds
- 2 tablespoons soy sauce
- 1 tablespoon sesame oil
- 2 tablespoons olive oil
- 3 cloves garlic, minced
- 1 tablespoon fresh ginger, grated
- 1 tablespoon honey or maple syrup
- 1 teaspoon rice vinegar
- Red pepper flakes (optional, for heat)
- Salt and pepper to taste
- Sesame seeds and chopped green onions for garnish

Instructions:

1. In a wok or large skillet, heat olive oil over medium-high heat.
2. Add minced garlic and grated ginger, sautéing for 1-2 minutes until fragrant.
3. Add broccoli florets to the wok and stir-fry for 3-4 minutes until they begin to soften but are still vibrant green.
4. In a small bowl, mix soy sauce, sesame oil, honey or maple syrup, rice vinegar, and red pepper flakes if using.
5. Pour the sauce over the broccoli and toss to coat evenly.

6. Add sliced almonds to the wok and continue to stir-fry for an additional 2-3 minutes until the broccoli is tender-crisp, and the almonds are toasted.
7. Season with salt and pepper to taste.
8. Garnish with sesame seeds and chopped green onions before serving.

Benefits:

- **Broccoli:** High in fiber, vitamins C and K, and antioxidants.
- **Almonds:** Provide healthy fats, protein, and essential nutrients.
- **Soy Sauce:** Adds savory flavor and contributes to the dish's umami profile.
- **Sesame Oil:** Adds a rich, nutty flavor and aroma.
- **Garlic and Ginger:** Add depth of flavor and may have immune-boosting properties.
- **Honey or Maple Syrup:** Adds sweetness to balance the savory and nutty elements.
- **Rice Vinegar:** Provides a tangy element.

Application:

- **Side Dish:** Serve as a flavorful and nutritious side dish alongside grilled chicken, fish, or tofu.

- **Vegetarian Main Course:** Enjoy as a satisfying vegetarian main course, served over rice or noodles.
- **Meal Prep:** Prepare a batch for meal prep and enjoy throughout the week.
- **Asian Fusion Dish:** Incorporate into Asian-inspired bowls or wraps for a quick and tasty meal.
- **Quick Weeknight Dinner:** Perfect for a speedy and healthful dinner option during busy weekdays.

Turmeric Grilled Chicken

Ingredients:
- 4 boneless, skinless chicken breasts
- 2 tablespoons olive oil
- 1 tablespoon ground turmeric
- 1 teaspoon ground cumin
- 1 teaspoon paprika
- 1 teaspoon garlic powder
- 1 teaspoon onion powder
- Salt and black pepper to taste
- Fresh cilantro or parsley for garnish (optional)
- Lemon wedges for serving

Instructions:
1. In a bowl, mix together olive oil, ground turmeric, ground cumin, paprika, garlic

powder, onion powder, salt, and black pepper to create the marinade.
2. Place the chicken breasts in a resealable plastic bag or shallow dish, and coat them evenly with the turmeric marinade. Seal the bag or cover the dish and refrigerate for at least 30 minutes, or ideally, marinate overnight for maximum flavor.
3. Preheat the grill to medium-high heat.
4. Remove the chicken from the marinade, letting excess drip off, and place them on the preheated grill.
5. Grill the chicken for 6-8 minutes per side or until the internal temperature reaches 165°F (74°C) and the chicken is no longer pink in the center.
6. Let the grilled chicken rest for a few minutes before slicing.
7. Garnish with fresh cilantro or parsley, and serve with lemon wedges.

Benefits:
- **Chicken:** A lean source of protein, rich in essential amino acids.
- **Turmeric:** Contains curcumin, known for its anti-inflammatory and antioxidant properties.
- **Cumin:** Adds a warm and earthy flavor and may aid in digestion.
- **Paprika:** Provides a mild, smoky flavor and adds a vibrant color.

- **Garlic and Onion Powder:** Enhance the overall flavor without added bulk.
- **Olive Oil:** Adds moisture to the chicken and provides healthy monounsaturated fats.

Application:

- **Main Course:** Serve Turmeric Grilled Chicken as the main dish for a flavorful and healthful meal.
- **Meal Prep:** Prepare a batch for meal prep and use throughout the week in salads, wraps, or bowls.
- **BBQ or Picnic:** Ideal for outdoor gatherings, adding a unique twist to your barbecue menu.
- **Protein Bowl:** Slice and incorporate into protein bowls with grains and vegetables.
- **Sandwiches or Wraps:** Use the grilled chicken as a filling for sandwiches or wraps.

Quinoa and Vegetable Salad

Ingredients:

- 1 cup quinoa, rinsed
- 2 cups water or vegetable broth
- 1 cup cherry tomatoes, halved
- 1 cucumber, diced
- 1 bell pepper (any color), diced

- 1/2 red onion, finely chopped
- 1/4 cup Kalamata olives, sliced
- 1/4 cup feta cheese, crumbled
- 1/4 cup fresh parsley, chopped
- 2 tablespoons olive oil
- 1 tablespoon balsamic vinegar
- 1 teaspoon Dijon mustard
- Salt and pepper to taste
- Lemon wedges for serving

Instructions:

1. In a saucepan, combine quinoa and water or vegetable broth. Bring to a boil, then reduce heat to low, cover, and simmer for 15-20 minutes or until quinoa is cooked and water is absorbed.
2. Fluff the quinoa with a fork and let it cool to room temperature.
3. In a large bowl, combine the cooked quinoa, cherry tomatoes, cucumber, bell pepper, red onion, Kalamata olives, feta cheese, and fresh parsley.
4. In a small bowl, whisk together olive oil, balsamic vinegar, Dijon mustard, salt, and pepper to create the dressing.
5. Pour the dressing over the quinoa and vegetable mixture and toss well to coat.
6. Allow the salad to chill in the refrigerator for at least 30 minutes to let the flavors meld.

7. Before serving, garnish with additional fresh parsley and serve with lemon wedges.

Benefits:
- **Quinoa:** A complete protein source, high in fiber, and rich in vitamins and minerals.
- **Vegetables:** Packed with vitamins, minerals, and antioxidants, supporting overall health.
- **Olives:** Provide healthy monounsaturated fats and add a savory flavor.
- **Feta Cheese:** Adds a creamy texture and contributes calcium and protein.
- **Olive Oil:** Healthy monounsaturated fats, supporting heart health.
- **Balsamic Vinegar:** Adds a sweet and tangy flavor, and may have potential health benefits.
- **Dijon Mustard:** Adds a zesty kick and is low in calories.

Application:
- **Main Dish:** Serve Quinoa and Vegetable Salad as a light and satisfying main course.
- **Side Dish:** Complement grilled chicken, fish, or other proteins with this vibrant salad.
- **Lunch Salad:** Enjoy a generous portion as a wholesome standalone lunch.
- **Potluck or Gathering:** A colorful and refreshing contribution to gatherings.
- **Meal Prep:** Prepare ahead for a quick and nutritious lunch option throughout the week.

CONCLUSION

As your completion "From Seed to Plate Cookbook: Recipes for Breast Cancer Resilience," we want to express our heartfelt appreciation to every reader who has joined us on this culinary and wellness journey.

This book arose from a common desire to inspire and elevate, recognizing that the route to recovery is a multifaceted quest that includes not just medical interventions but also the caring embrace of nutrition and culinary care.

We wanted to make more than just a collection of foods with these recipes. We hoped to foster a holistic approach to well-being that recognized the interdependence of body, mind, and spirit. Each dish is an expression of love, care, and the conviction that every decision we make in the kitchen contributes to our total vitality.

We hope that once you shut this book, you will carry the sense of resilience featured on each page with you. May the aromas remain on your mouth, reminding you of your inner power.

Remember that cooking a nutritious meal is an affirmation—an affirmation of life, health, and the unshakeable spirit that pulls us onward.

Allow this culinary adventure to instill a greater appreciation for the food on your plate, the gardens that provide its bounty, and the transformational power of your own kitchen.

May these dishes continue to be companions on your route to recovery, demonstrating that wellbeing is a constant, changing journey rather than a destination.

Finally, we want to thank you for your bravery, courage, and dedication to wellbeing. May the tastes endure, the memories nourish, and the road to resilience be filled with joy.

May your route from Seed to plate be strewn with love, healing, and the profound beauty of a life well-lived.